HOW TO LOSE WEIGHT PERMANENTLY:

An Inference from Brain Research for Long-Term Weight Loss

By

JOCELYN SMITH

Copy right © by JOCELYN SMITH 2023. All rights reserved

Before this document is duplicated or repro
 manner, the publisher's consent must be gained.

How to Lose Weight Permanently

Table of Contents

Introduction

Energy expenditure must be greater than calorie intake to cause weight growth. But as is covered in this book, a complicated web of interactions between genetic, behavioral, and environmental factors leads to being overweight or obese. Although the overweight public has access to thousands, if not hundreds, of weight-loss programs, diets, treatments, and devices, it is challenging for experts, researchers, and those who are overweight to develop long-term, efficient weight-loss and maintenance plans during to the complex causes of obesity.

Only 1 to 3 percent of people who successfully lose weight can keep it off in the long run, according to estimates.

The effectiveness and safety of numerous weight loss strategies are examined in this book, as well as the combinations of tactics that seem to be linked to successful weight loss. The elements of good weight maintenance will also be studied because it may be harder to maintain weight decrease, which could worsen the obesity problem. There is also a brief discussion of potential public policy initiatives to combat obesity and offer assistance to people who are seeking to lose weight or maintain their weight.

Chapter 1

Why Does Your Body Want Food?

You should expect to feel hungry if you go several hours without consuming because your body needs food for energy. However, if your stomach constantly grumbles, even after consuming, your health may be in trouble.

Polyphagia is the medical term for severe appetite. Consult your doctor if you constantly feel famished. Numerous factors can result in persistent hunger.

Diabetes

The sugar in food is converted by your body into a fuel called glucose. Diabetes, however, prevents glucose from reaching your cells.

Your body signals you to consume more by making you excrete it instead. Particularly those with type 1 diabetes may ingest enormous amounts of food while still losing weight. In addition to a rise in appetite, diabetes symptoms might include: Extreme thirst, the urge to urinate more frequently, unexplained weight loss, hazy eyesight, slow-healing wounds and bruises, tingling or soreness in your hands or feet, and fatigue are all symptoms of excessive thirst.

Reduced Blood Sugar

When the level of glucose in your blood declines to extremely low levels, you experience hypoglycemia. People with diabetes frequently fret about it, but it can also result from other medical conditions.

Hepatitis, kidney conditions, insulinomas, neuroendocrine tumors of the pancreas, and issues with the pituitary or adrenal organs are a few of them. People with hypoglycemia may appear inebriated in severe circumstances. They can have difficulties walking and speech slurred.

Additional indications can include:Anxiety symptoms include: *Pale skin* *Shaking* *Sweating* *Tingling in the mouth* *Feeling like your heart is missing a beat*

Unable to slumber

The hormones in your body that regulate hunger might be impacted by not receiving enough sleep. People who are sleep deprived have larger appetites and struggle to feel satisfied after consuming.

When you're weary, you're also more inclined to pursue items that are heavy in fat and calories.

Other consequences of inadequate slumber include: An inability to stay awake during the day, a change in mood, clumsiness, more accidents, difficulty staying awake, and weight gain.

Stress

Your body releases the hormone cortisol when you're anxious or agitated. This intensifies how famished you feel.

Many anxious people often want foods that are heavy in fat, sugar, or both. It might be an attempt by your body to "shut off" the area of your brain that makes you apprehensive.

Additional indicators include:*Exclamations of fury *Fatigue *Headache *Sleep issues *Upset stomach

Diet

Foods don't all satiate you in the same manner. The foods that best satiate hunger are those that are high in fiber or protein, such as lean meats, fish, or dairy products. Fruits, vegetables, whole grains, and legumes are excellent sources of fiber.

Your cholesterol levels can be reduced by consuming healthy fats such as those found in nuts, salmon, and sunflower oil.

They're essential to a balanced diet and can increase your sense of fullness after eating.

While lacking essential nutrients, white bread, many prepared meals, fast food, and pastries are heavy in fat and unhealthful carbohydrates. If you consume a lot of these, you can experience post-meal appetite. It's conceivable that you overate.

If you consume slower and chew your food thoroughly, as opposed to eating it quickly, you might find that you feel more satisfied after a meal. It can also be beneficial to focus on what is on your plate rather than the TV or your phone.

Medication

Some medicines may cause you to feel more famished than usual. This is a well-known property of antihistamines, which are used to treat allergies, as well as SSRI antidepressants, steroids, several diabetic medications, and antipsychotic medications.

If you've put on weight since commencing your medication, the prescription may be causing you to feel hungry. Find out from your doctor what additional medications might be effective for you.

Pregnancy

Pregnant women often report a significant increase in appetite. Your body does this to make sure the baby has access to enough nutrients to thrive.

The average woman gains 1 pound each week during the second and third trimesters, and between 4 and 6 pounds during the first three months (your doctor will refer to this as the first trimester).

Other indicators that you may be pregnant include: *A missing period *A constant need to urinate *An unsettled stomach *Sore breasts or enlarged breasts.

How Frequently You Workout

When you exercise, your body burns calories for sustenance. Your metabolism, or the way your body burns energy, is enhanced as a result. That may contribute to an increase in hunger in some people.

Chapter2

Why your Emotions constantly makes you crave for food

When you're unhappy or down, do you immediately head to the pantry? Nobody is excluding you. When enduring intensely painful feelings, it's common for people to turn to food for solace. When you eat as a reaction to your feelings, it is emotional eating. It happens to everyone occasionally.

Our bodies need nutrition to survive. Eating should make you feel better since it triggers the reward system in the brain. It might become an issue if you frequently overeat emotionally and don't have any other coping techniques.

In those situations, eating may seem like a coping mechanism, but it doesn't deal with the underlying problem. If you're anxious, stressed, bored, lonely, depressed, or fatigued, food won't make you feel better.

Some people experience guilt and shame as a result of their pattern of using food as a coping mechanism, which are harder feelings to manage.

You may feel hungry in almost any situation.

The following are some outside factors that can contribute to emotional eating: *work stress* *financial worries* *health concerns* *relationship troubles*

Emotional eating is more likely among people who follow rigid diets or have a history of dieting.

Lack of introspective awareness (not being aware of how you feel), alexithymia (the inability to understand, process, or explain emotions), and emotion dysregulation (the inability to control emotions) are other potential internal reasons.

The underactive cortisol response to stress (Hypothalamic Pituitary Adrenal, or HPA) In many cases, emotional eating becomes a habit. The behavior becomes more ingrained the more food is used to cope.

Chapter3

How to Determine REAL Hunger

Physical hunger symptoms can differ from person to person, and some people have spent a long time ignoring their natural hunger cues and are no longer aware of what those cues look like. Furthermore, long-term calorie restriction can slow metabolism, resulting in hunger even when not losing weight.

This could be the case for you if you've spent a lot of time restricting yourself.

If this is the case, it is best to consult with a dietician, nutritionist, or therapist who specializes in this area. *Growing stomach *Low energy *Headache *Dizziness *Difficulty focusing *Shakiness

How to Use Hunger Indicators

According to studies, the majority of weight-loss programs fail. When your body is deprived of calories, your metabolism often slows, and your hunger increases. Eating in response to hunger signals can be more effective for weight maintenance, but it may not always be effective for weight loss.

Learning to use your hunger and satiety signals more mindfully can help you understand when to eat and when you may be seeking the comfort of food for other reasons.

Detecting Your Hunger Cues

*Take a moment to consider whether you are physically hungry. Examine your entire body from head to toe to ascertain your temperament and physical condition.

*Eat slowly to allow your body time to detect fullness.

Eating by Feeling

Understanding hunger and fullness cues to help guide eating decisions is one of the most important principles of intuitive eating. This eating style can assist people in learning how to balance a healthy weight and lifestyle with their dietary choices. Respecting your body's biological hunger signals is one of the most important aspects of intuitive eating.

A scale can be used to effectively honor your hunger and fullness cues. Eat whenever your hunger level reaches 3 or 4, and never let it fall below 3.

Eating when you are extremely hungry can impair your ability to select foods that will help you meet your needs to the greatest extent possible. Furthermore, hunger hormones are released in greater quantities, increasing your hunger and possibly leading to overeating.

When you reach level 6, you should reduce or stop eating. Allow your body to send fullness cues after 15 to 20 minutes to see if you are still ravenous. Often, after waiting, you will feel full but not claustrophobic. If you're still hungry, consume until you reach level 7.

Chapter4

Weight Loss Challenges And Their Solutions

There is no one method that works for everyone when it comes to losing weight, according to recent studies. The biggest determining factor in whether you are successful in losing weight is you. Poor diet, inactivity, genetics, medications, and other aspects of your lifestyle and surroundings can all affect your ability to lose weight.

However, certain physiological situations exaggerate the significance of particular weight loss strategies.

Because of this, it's crucial to concentrate your efforts on the things that will help you get the most for your money.

As with most things, adding more tactics might result in further weight reduction as you start to see results and the pounds start to come off. Here is a fast tutorial on how to lose weight while dealing with some typical life obstacles; maybe one of them relates to you.

Challenge 1: As people age, they eat more for a variety of reasons. The biggest one is a drop in physical activity.

Less movement causes more calories to be stored as fat in the body as opposed to being turned into energy for activities.

Additionally, a slower metabolism results from the fact that we gradually lose muscle mass as we age – up to 3-5% after age 30 if you're inactive.

Solution: Strength training can assist create new muscle and stop the loss of muscular mass.

They burn more calories because muscle cells have a far higher metabolic activity than fat cells.

Your metabolism is increased when your muscle mass increases.

How to Lose Weight Permanently

To increase strength without damaging yourself, start slowly and warm up before exercising.

Start with two sessions each week of 10 repetitions each of eight to ten different exercises for the upper, lower, and core. Use 5- to 10-pound dumbbells for other workouts and your own body weight for pushups and pullups.

At the end of each exercise, you should feel as though you can only perform one or two more reps; if you can, it's time to increase the weight.

Challenge 2: One of the most difficult aspects of being a new mother is probably losing baby weight while being exhausted from having a newborn. Women of ordinary weight are advised to gain 25 to 35 pounds on average, although many end up gaining more. The majority of women lose about 10-15 pounds in the first week following delivery, but the remainder can take longer.

Solution: New mothers should engage in a healthy level of physical exercise (once they have recovered from giving birth) and eat a balanced diet, especially if they plan to breastfeed.

How to Lose Weight Permanently

Light aerobic exercise is a terrific method to improve your mood and start losing the additional weight you put on initially (be sure your doctor has given the go-ahead).

Plus, you may bring the baby, making it a great pastime for strengthening your relationship. Start with 1-2 miles of pram walks when your doctor gives the all-clear. According to the Centres for Disease Control and Prevention, a 154-pound person may burn about 230 calories in just 30 minutes of walking at 4.5 miles per hour.

Challenge 3: Despite eating the same meal as someone with a normal metabolism, someone with a lower basal metabolism will use less energy. Worse still, you don't want to exercise because of the exhaustion brought on by a slow metabolism.

Solution: It's crucial to get your thyroid examined if you think you might have a slower metabolism than average. The right drug regimen can significantly impact how well hypothyroidism patients are able to raise their activity level and lose weight.

While high-intensity interval training may seem challenging at first, research indicates that it may be able to increase metabolism.

Short bursts of all-out effort are interspersed with recovery periods throughout this kind of workout. Three times each week, the American College of Sports Medicine advises performing 3-5 sets of 30-second sprints, followed by 4-4.5 minutes of rest (be sure to warm up and cool down).

Challenge 4: Hypoglycemia, often known as low blood sugar, can make you feel weak, tired, and headachey. Being physically active is made more difficult by these factors, which frequently results in weight gain and the inability to lose additional pounds. Fortunately, the same dietary modifications that can significantly impact blood sugar regulation also help people lose weight.

Solution: Limiting your intake of sugar and fat will assist control your blood sugar levels while also making you forgo some of the worst junk food choices.

Increase your intake of complex carbs with low glycemic index, soluble fiber-rich meals, and lean protein-rich foods such steel-cut oats, whole-grain pasta, almonds, fish, apples, and eggplant.

Challenge 5: As you become older, not only does your metabolism slow down, but you also don't burn calories as effectively as you once did.This implies that many people gain weight as they reach middle age, even those who have never had a weight problem before.

Solution: To maintain weight over the long term, middle-aged women needed to clock an average of 60 minutes of moderate-intensity activity, according to research published in the Journal of the American Medical Association. Despite the fact that this is twice the usual recommendation of 30 minutes per day, other study demonstrates the value of aerobic exercise for middle-aged persons in terms of weight loss and general health.

This can involve going for a walk, running, swimming, cycling, or using the elliptical machine.

Challenge 6: Everything from your appetite to your energy levels can be impacted when hormones like cortisol, testosterone, and leptin aren't working as they should. It may seem impossible to lose weight as a result.

Solution: While researchers continue to explore possible solutions, making lifestyle and nutritional adjustments can help balance your hormones, which can increase energy and reduce cravings. To find out if you're getting the correct balance of nutrients, start by tracking your dietary intake using the MyFitnessPal app.

Make dietary alterations based on your unique circumstances, which might assist in identifying the cause of the issue.

Another area of your daily life that needs your attention is sleep. According to research, when you don't receive enough of it, you seek additional foods high in fat and carbohydrates. Leptin levels in your blood will be balanced out by getting enough sleep, which will help you stop cravings.

Chapter5

Get Yourself A Distinctive Eating Plan

A wise food plan is necessary to lose weight in a healthy and long-lasting way. Your body needs the right amount of calories and nutrition for sustained energy during workouts and daily activities. The secret to losing weight and keeping it off over time is to keep that balance.

A convenient and delicious menu is included in a healthy meal plan for weight loss that includes all the vitamins and minerals your body requires to maintain energy and build muscle.

Develop a weight-loss diet plan that supports your lifestyle, goals, and habits by following these steps.

STEP ONE: REFRAIN FROM USING CALORIE-COUNTING DIETS.

Typical diet plans establish a daily calorie target. Dieters are advised to keep their daily caloric intake to a certain range and eat meals that are complete with all the nutrients they require to stay alive.

However, this fundamental notion dooms a lot of dieters to failure before they even start. We recommend a different strategy than calorie counting.

How to Lose Weight Permanently

Why is counting calories daily the wrong way to think about dietary intake?

Every food has a unique range of calories. It becomes difficult to maintain strict tracking of your intake unless you eat nearly the same thing every day.

There are many occasions, such as going out with friends or going on vacation, when dieters simply cannot keep up a strict daily count without giving up the enjoyment of those activities.

*A "cheat day" is a day when the dieter is allowed to eat whatever they want without counting calories to avoid temptation.

Due to one weekly day of overindulgence, it is possible to follow a daily restrictive calorie restriction and still fail to lose weight. Calorie counting each day seems to encourage undereating. Dieters strive to stay within their restrictions to maintain calorie deficits. Too many calories missed hurt weight loss efforts over time.

Instead of limiting your daily caloric intake, we advise you to create a diet plan that meets all of your nutritional needs to maintain a healthy lifestyle. Because it boosts energy levels, is less restrictive, and gives you the freedom to eat whatever you want in moderation, this technique is very effective for weight loss programs.

How to Lose Weight Permanently

Everybody's nutritional requirements are different depending on their age, weight, level of exercise, and other medical factors. You have the freedom to eat a variety of foods to achieve your weight loss objectives when you set these nutritional goals or standards.

These dietary objectives concentrate on the amounts of protein, carbohydrates, fats, vitamins, and minerals you consume. A more effective method for weight loss than counting calories is maintaining these vital components in balance with what your body needs.

STEP TWO: EXERCISE YOUR MACROS

Dieting is about more than just how much you eat. For your body to build muscle, burn fat, and maintain a high level of energy, you must also make sure that you're giving it what it needs.

Macronutrients are the fundamental building blocks that your body needs to carry out these tasks. Your main source of calories comes from these fundamental nutrients. There are three main types of macros:

*Carbohydrates. The body breaks down both simple and complex sugar chains to create energy for the muscles.

*Fats. When quick-burning carbohydrates are not available, extra calories are stored in fat cells to provide emergency energy. Numerous hormonal and cognitive processes depend heavily on fat.

*Proteins. The body's tissues can develop and repair themselves with the help of these powerful macros, which provide sustainable energy and materials.

You have the best chance of achieving your ideal body while avoiding feeling constrained or worn out if you balance these macronutrients.

According to conventional wisdom, you should split your daily caloric intake into 35% healthy fat, 40% protein, and 25% carbohydrates. To determine your ideal combination, use an online calculator for a more customized ratio.

STEP THREE: FIND FOODS THAT FIT.

Once you are aware of how much food you require, take some time to select meals that go well with your new way of life. Meals that you'll eat are a requirement of a successful weight loss diet plan.

How to Lose Weight Permanently

You're less likely to follow your plan if you don't enjoy the food you're eating.

It's essential to put some effort into exploring new menu options, though. Due to a restrictive diet high in empty calories, weight loss programs are frequently used by dieters.

Building a long-term eating plan requires you to increase the number of healthy food options in your daily diet.

Make a list of the foods and ingredients you enjoy the most to start. Once you start eating healthy, try to increase your intake of one or two additional fruits, vegetables, or grains each week.

It's useful to include information on the macronutrient value of each item because doing so will enable you to choose how much of each you should eat at each meal.

STEP FOUR: BUY RECIPES IN ADVANCE

You can now begin gathering a variety of recipes that use the foods you are allowed to eat. Pay close attention to the preparation guidelines. The amount of macronutrients in your food depends greatly on how you cook it.

How to Lose Weight Permanently

Your diet plan for weight loss must include a wide variety of recipes to keep you from getting bored. The main reason many dieters fail to reach their objectives is that they grow bored with their daily menus. You'll always look forward to your next meal if there is variety on the menu. An excellent way to store your recipes is in an online recipe book.

If you do enough research, you can tailor your recipe collection to your tastes. Are sweetbreads and pastries your favorite foods? Discover low-calorie variations of your preferred baked goods.

Are sauces an essential part of your typical mealtime? Look for homemade versions of the condiments you use the most frequently.

Do you feel anxious about the idea of giving up fried foods? Look for recipes that use your oven to replicate the desired crunchiness without adding extra fat.

Make a list of the restaurants you go to the most often if you're someone who always has to be on the go. Inquire about the menu items' nutritional information from the staff. Create a list of options that fit within your dietary budget using the data from that analysis.

STEP FIVE: SET A SCHEDULE FOR EATING

Just as crucial as what you eat is when you eat. Every day, our bodies go through cycles that make it harder for us to process the contents of our stomachs.

Additionally, your current health conditions or adjustments to how your body functions can affect how you process food.

A diet plan for weight loss that adheres to the conventional paradigm of three meals per day often fails. This is particularly valid for people who drastically reduce their daily caloric intake. Consider spacing your meals and snacks out by about three hours.

How to Lose Weight Permanently

This prevents you from becoming excessively hungry and turning to unhealthy options to satisfy your hunger.

Here are some useful hints to assist you in creating the ideal diet strategy for weight loss.

*Eat a hearty dinner to reduce late-night snacking. Within an hour of waking up, eat a high-protein breakfast.

*Follow your established eating schedule.

Consult your doctor for assistance in creating a plan that helps maintain the proper blood sugar levels if you have diabetes or other glucose conditions that are affected by your eating habits.

STEP SIX: TRACK, ANALYZE, AND MAKE ADJUSTMENTS

To keep track of your meal plan, use a food diary. This creates a record that enables you to look over your eating patterns and gauge how well your plan is working. Make adjustments as necessary to maintain your progress toward your ideal weight. Never be afraid to switch things up if an eating regimen isn't producing the desired results.

Chapter6

Make The Weight Loss Permanent

Now that you've attained the magic number, what do you do? The goal is to get rid of the additional weight and make sure it never reappears. Regrettably, only around one-third of dieters can maintain their weight reduction. Those who have lost weight successfully are aware that doing so needs attention, which for some people might be more difficult than simply reducing the weight. You must alter your way of life to keep the weight off.

If you pick up the previous behaviors that caused you to become overweight in the first place, weight gain will unavoidably happen. Maintaining a good diet and consistent exercise habits is essential for long-term weight reduction, just like you did while you were losing weight. Many people relax their guard when they lose weight and then gain it back. You can take a brief but essential rest when you're done, Below are few tips that can help you maintain a permanent Weight Loss.

Practice makes perfect

The more you do something, the easier it gets. It takes time to incorporate such good behaviors into a routine. Don't allow all your hard work to go to waste, and be gentle to yourself. Be prepared and conscious of your weaknesses. You'll be tempted by particular meals and circumstances, but if you remain steadfast in your determination, you can withstand temptations. Moderation is an excellent tactic in those challenging situations.

Pick a day of the week when you can give yourself a little indulgence. One of my favorite methods for keeping weight off is this.

Otherwise, you can have unanticipated events that cause you to have more than one "off" day every week.

Every week must provide a new version of this day. I permit myself to indulge in little amounts of my favorite foods on my designated day off, which is typically a Saturday for obvious reasons. However, you should only have a tiny portion of the cheesecake.

It is essentially cheating that has been reined in. It works wonders for me; you might find it helpful as well. Knowing that I can relax on Saturday keeps me on top of things during the week.

Victorious losers

Successful weight-loss individuals can act as role models for us. Before a person is registered with the National Weight Control Registry (NWCR), at least 60 pounds must be dropped and kept off-limits for at least five years. They carry out the following tasks:

It has to be highlighted. Keeping a meal journal is a fantastic tool to assist you in staying on track. Eat gently and healthfully. The majority of successful losers follow low-fat diets because diet gimmicks, specialist foods, or cure-all medications don't work over the long term.

*Everyday physical exercise. These folks regard walking to be their favorite form of exercise and incorporate it into their daily routine in the same way they would wash their teeth. Participants in the NWCR exercise for roughly one hour each day.

*Start the day off right with breakfast. All studies support a healthy morning routine. Check your weight frequently. They change their diet and exercise routine as soon as they put on a few pounds to get back to a healthy weight. According to James O. Hill, Ph.D., of the NWCR, the longer people maintain their weight reduction, the easier it is to sustain the decrease.

Living a healthy lifestyle is no longer a hardship in the new lives of successful losers. It should be a way of life rather than a diet.

It does get simpler to maintain a healthy weight with time. If you can make it two years, there's a good chance you're safe.

Remain devoted

Keep your motivation strong and don't allow failures to stop you from moving forward: Simply go back on the right course if you stray from it by picking yourself up.

If you can get your brain to think and act like a skinny person, you can stay that way for the rest of your life.

And it becomes easier the more you do it. By the time you get to the maintenance stage, you probably already have habits, tactics, and abilities that have kept you on track. Take pleasure. You deserve praise for implementing healthy eating and exercise habits that not only motivate your loved ones but also significantly improve your health.

According to studies, long-term weight maintenance is correlated with keeping in touch with the people or programs that helped you lose weight. It makes sense to stay in touch with the people who gave you your initial push to success. We'll help you keep the weight off if you stick with us!